GSH (GLUTATHIONE)

A Secret

To a Longer and Better Life

By Dr.Neo

FOREWARD

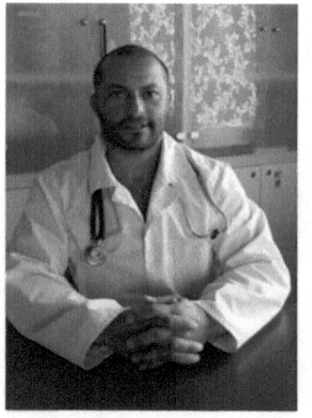

Dr. Neo, a successful holistic medicine practitioner, has come up with his new book "**A Secret to a Longer and Better Life**" for those who are interested to know how to live a healthier and a happier life.

Although many books and articles had been written on this marvellous substance called Glutathione, Dr. Neos's book offers a more readable treatment of the subject that can be appreciated by health professionals and laypeople alike.

Dr. Neo is a staunch advocate of bringing health consciousness to a greater number of people. In "**A Secret to a Longer and Better Life**", he discusses many of the well-known (as well as not-so-well-known) facts about Glutathione that play a big part in the health and well-being of people. He has written this book in such a way that it could be appreciated and students and by readers who merely seek additional knowledge about the topic like homemakers and lay health enthusiasts.

Dr. Neo bases this book on his personal knowledge and experiences as a medical practitioner. He combines these with the latest findings of medical experts in the field of nutrition on Glutathione. He explains the seeming complexities of this substance in clearer terms and debunks old myths about it, thus assuring his readers of updated information on the subject.

With his book "**A Secret to a Longer and Better Life**", Dr. Neo is able to attain his goal of advocating holistic health care by highlighting the important role this substance plays in maintaining a person's well-being.

Dr. Neo dedicates this book to <u>you</u>, his readers, and wishes you all good health now and through the years to come!

TABLE OF CONTENTS

Titles   **Page**

COPYRIGHT

INTRODUCTION

This book, "**GSH (Glutathione) --- A Secret to a Longer and Better Life**", discusses in detail **Glutathione**, a remarkable but often ignored substance that enables the body to function properly.

What we are going to learn from this book is the importance of Glutathione in our life and how this knowledge can increase our faith in fighting any disease.

Remember that you are your best doctor!

BRIEF EXPLANATION ON THE IMPORTANCE OF GLUTATHIONE IN THE BODY

Glutathione is a protein (3-peptide) and its main work is to <u>aid</u> in the regulation of the 3 main functions in the body (best remembered for the acronym A.I.D.)

A stands for Antioxidant

I stands for Immune System

D stands for Detoxification.

Some Facts about the Glutathione:

- Protein is produced within each cell of human and animal body and is the main component that keeps us healthy.

- It is made up of 3 amino-acids, namely: Cysteine, Glycine and Glutamate.

- The level of Glutathione in our cells is predictive of how long we will live.

- It plays a crucial role in the regulation of many body functions required to sustain life. No other antioxidant is as imperative to overall health as Glutathione.

- Approximately 50% of the body's Glutathione production depends largely on the consumption of fruits and vegetables. Unfortunately, modern technology, with its introduction of pesticides and genetically modified foods (GMO), has depleted exponentially these natural food sources and thus compromising their availability.

  This results in the very limited amount of Glutathione derived from these foods in reaching the bloodstream, considering that most of it is lost in the digestive tract. The need, therefore, of our body for Glutathione production has risen dramatically increased while its ability to produce it naturally has diminished considerably.

BENEFITS OF GLUTATHIONE

Dr. Jimmy Gutman considers Glutathione as the **master antioxidant** because without it, none of the other antioxidants, like Vitamin C and E, can function properly.

- **In the Immune System**: This system is set to protect our body from things that are not supposed to be there. These refer to any microbial and even tumour cells. Our body is developing potential tumour cells every day and the Immune System is always on the alert to keep us healthy 24/7.

  Anyone with compromised or weak immune system is susceptible to contracting all the diseases, even cancer. Glutathione is the main component that can keep the white blood cells and lymphoid cells clean from toxins so they can function properly. These blood cells need sufficient amount of Glutathione inside them to keep them healthy to fight any threat to our health.

- In **Detoxification**, liver is the mother organ for detoxification and the body's most concentrated source of Glutathione is found in the liver. Glutathione detoxifies the liver by getting rid of all the toxins, heavy metals and free radicals from this organ. Clinical evidence shows that low glutathione levels is linked with many common illnesses as well as diseases of aging. The quality of the detoxification in the liver will decide whether we get sick or not.

In his book "GSH Your Body's Most Powerful Protector", Dr. Jimmy Gutman covers all the necessary information on Glutathione. Thanks to him, that through his book, we have gained an even greater understanding and appreciation of this substance that he refers to as the Mother of Antioxidants.

PROPERTIES OF GLUTATHIONE

DNA SYNTHESIS AND REPAIR

Glutathione is useful for the repair and synthesis of **DNA, proteins, amino acid transport,** and **enzyme activation**. The proper synthesis of DNA helps mitochondria to function properly and converts food into **ATP** (energy fuel). A sufficient level of Glutathione in the body ensures the proper functioning of the cell by providing energy and getting rid of any harmful substances like toxins, heavy metals, oxidative stress and free radicals.

REGULATION OF CELL GROWTH AND DIVISION

Hydrogen Peroxide (H_2O_2) is the number one killer of any pathogen and cancerous cell. Unfortunately, its presence prevents division and growth in the normal cells. Glutathione is capable of converting Hydrogen Peroxide into harmless **water (H_2O).**

PROTEIN SYNTHESIS

Glutathione can maintain proteins in their proper form. With its sulfur atom, it is able to react with unnatural sulfur-sulfur bonds in proteins, breaking them and allowing the proper pairings to form.

AMINO ACID TRANSPORT

Since Glutathione is located predominately inside the cell, it has the ability to transport substances like amino acids, in and out of the cell

ENZYME CATALYSIS AND ACTIVATION

Glutathione is responsible for the chemical reactions between some enzymes and changing their forms to reduced state, or change them from one state to another. Also the highly reactive sulfide bond, has the ability to activate enzymes to move from one phase to the next.

METABOLISM OF HARMFUL AGENTS

In the liver, the enzyme glutathione S-transferase takes the sulfur from glutathione and attaches it to any toxic molecules and heavy metals. This makes them more soluble to water and transported to the elimination systems to be excreted from the body. In the case of carcinogens, Glutathione transforms them to non-genotoxic compounds so they can be eliminated without causing damage to any cell or DNA.

RECYCLING OF OTHER ANTIOXIDANTS

Glutathione has the ability to restore oxidized alpha-lipoic acid, vitamin C and vitamin E to their active state by donating them the missing electron needed. That is why Glutathione is called the mother of all antioxidants.

LIVER

Liver is the mother organ where most processing of foods occurs for the proper functioning of the body. The highest concentration, therefore, of Glutathione is found in the liver. It aids in the detoxifying process (which inhibits the aging process and prevents diseases), protects the liver from damage and repairs damaged liver cells. Glutathione also helps to prevent chronic inflammation that leads to free radical formation and oxidative damage. Oxidative damage speeds up the signs of aging.

BLOOD-BRAIN BARRIER

What is **blood-brain barrier** and what is its correlation with Glutathione? Blood-brain barrier is a barrier that prevents large substances from entering the brain and damages it. Normally, the endothelial tissue of the capillaries (the smallest blood vessels where the exchange of substances occur from blood to cells and vice versa) has small spaces between each individual cell so substance can move readily between the inside and outside of the vessel. However, in the brain, the endothelial cells fit tightly together so substances cannot pass out from the bloodstream. The blood-brain barrier, together with antioxidants, prevents toxins and heavy metals (aluminium, mercury, lead, cadmium) from accumulating in the brain. The accumulation of these substances may cause severe damage (Multiple Sclerosis, ALS (Amyotrophic Lateral Sclerosis), Alzheimer's disease etc). Glutathione is one of these antioxidants that are capable of entering the blood-brain barrier and clear away these harmful toxins and heavy metals.

INFLAMMATION & NF-kB

What is **inflammation** and what is **NF-kB?** What is their correlation between them and Glutathione?

- **Inflammation** is a natural and healthy non-specific immune response. In medicine, according to PhD Neal Stewart Rote, inflammation belongs to the mechanism of self-defence. It is a biochemical and cellular process occurs in the vascularised tissues. Most of the essential components of the inflammatory process are found in the circulation. Most of the early mediators of inflammation affect the vascular bed by increasing the movement of plasma and blood cells in the circulation into the tissues surrounding the injury. These substances defend the host against infection and facilitate tissue repair and healing. When inflammation persists longer than necessary, it crosses the line between healthy and harmful.

Cellular Injury → acute inflammation → chronic inflammation → granuloma

                             Healing   Healing Healing

- **NF-kB (Nuclear Factor kappa Beta)** is a small protein complex that controls transcription of DNA, found in almost all human and animal cells and is involved in cellular responses to stimuli like stress, free radicals, pathogens etc. NF-kB is responsible for the proper formation of the healthy cell. Diachronic stress, psychosomatic issues, improper diet, heavy metals, alcohol etc. can cause incorrect regulation of DNA that may result to cancer, inflammation, autoimmune diseases etc.

Understanding the relationship between NF-kB and inflammation is critical to maintaining your health and longevity. NFkB is like a "smoke sensor". It detects dangerous threats and "turns on" the genes that produce inflammation that may cause severe damages in long term.

Very few nutrients are capable of switching the NF-kB off once it is turned on. Glutathione is one of them. Glutathione also repairs any oxidative damage caused by inflammation. Now you understand the importance of Glutathione to 99% of diseases.

IMMUNE SYSTEM

The immune system is an elegant and complex group of components that combine to fight disease, infections and various pathogens. A healthy immune system can quickly detect any invader and rapidly destroy it. A compromised immune system, on the other hand, allows invading organisms to flourish. The body's immune response relies on various white blood cells and natural barriers to block any invader. Glutathione boosts white blood cell production to fight invaders. These white blood cells are produced in the bone marrow and mature in the thymus gland, but are present in the blood and lymph nodes. These are called Lymphocytes T or T-cells.

T-cells are at the core of our immunity, and tailor the body's immune response to invaders. B-cell lymphocytes identify the unwanted invader from T-cells and release specific antibodies to the specific intruder. T-cells also have the ability to shut down the immune response when the job is done. Otherwise, they will make mistakes and start attacking the body itself.

These are referred to as allergies and autoimmune diseases. The immune system is responsible for anything happen in our body. Diachronic stress, psychosomatic issues, improper diet, heavy metals, alcohol etc. can deplete the immune system and then anything can occur, from cancer to any infectious or autoimmune response. Glutathione is important for keeping the immune system functioning properly.

RED BLOOD CELLS

According to Lubert Stryer of Stanford University, Reduced Glutathione (explained in the next chapter) is essential of maintaining the normal structure of red blood cells and for keeping haemoglobin in the ferrous state. Cells with lower level of Reduced Glutathione are more susceptible to haemolysis. Drugs such as pamaquine (used to treat malaria tears ago) distort the surface of red blood cells in the absence of Reduced Glutathione. This makes them more susceptible to destruction and removal by the spleen. These drugs also increase the rate of formation of toxic peroxides that are usually eliminated with their reaction to Reduced Glutathione.

REGULATION OF HOMOCYSTEINE

Homocysteine is a hologue of the amino acid Cysteine, differing by additional methylene bridge (CH_2). Homocysteine can be recycled into methionine or converted into cysteine with the aid of certain B-vitamins, enzymes and Glutathione. High levels of Homocysteine in the blood is the syndrome called '*hyperhomocysteinemia*' which can injure endothelial cells and result into atherosclerosis (hardening of blood vessels) that leads to coronary artery diseases like heart attack. The body uses a large amount of Glutathione to metabolize Homocysteine and convert it to useful amino acid, Cysteine, and prevent cell injury.

SKIN HEALTH AND SKIN COSMETICS

Glutathione presents in each cell in the body. It plays a major role in detoxifying our cells, by removing heavy metals, toxins and free radicals. All of which can damage our cells and their quality, including skin cells. Proper quantity of Glutathione in the body can help to improve the health of every cell, particularly apparent in the skin, hair and nails. The radiant glow it gives is a result of healthy cells and reduced toxicity in the body. Skin complexion, age spots and wrinkles can by limited by proper quantity of glutathione in our cells.

How can Glutathione improve the whitening of the skin? Glutathione helps to prevent activation of Tyrosinase by reducing free radicals in the body that can activate it and cause an increase in melanin production. Melanin is the pigment and pigment spots the give our skin its colour, produced by the activation of the enzyme Tyrosinase.

With Glutathione being so critical for keeping cells healthy, science went a step further and put it into cosmetic and personal care products. Skin cells are also subject to oxidative damage from exposure to ultraviolet light from the sun and from pollutants in the environment. At least half of sun-related skin damages are due to free radical formation such as skin aging, skin cancer, skin spots. These damages can be fixed by topical antioxidants like Glutathione, alpha-lipoic acid and Vitamin C.

Antioxidants like Glutathione have anti-inflammatory benefits so they can reduce skin inflammation after procedures like laser resurfacing.

Products like facial scrubs, moisturizers, anti-aging products, toners, exfoliating products and sunscreen, contain Glutathione.

Since Glutathione as a supplement is difficult to be taken orally due to stomach juices, so in cosmetics, it is available as cream, lotion, serum, gel, and liquid to the skin.

The Environmental Working Group's Skin Deep Databases classifies it as a low hazard cosmetic ingredient.

FORMS AND STRUCTURES OF GLUTATHIONE

Glutathione is the most biologically abundant low molecular weight intracellular thiol. By way of the reducing power of its free Sulfhydryl (-SH), it plays a key role in many cellular processes mentioned above. Glutahtione is synthesised intracellularly from its constituent amino acids by the consecutive action of two enzymes, γ-glutamylcysteine ligase (γ-GCL), previously known as γ-glutamylcysteine synthetase (γ-GCS), and glutathione synthetase (GS), with both reactions consuming ATP (energy):

L-glutamic acid +l-cysteine ──────────▸ γ-Glutaminecysteine (γ-GC)

    enzyme γ-GCS+ATP   + ADP

γ-GlutamineCysteine + Glycine ──────────▸ Glutathione

    enzyme GS+ATP   + ADP

γ-GlutamineCysteine, an unusual gamma-peptide bond, is resistant to most proteases. This means that oral delivery of GGC or γ-GC is not subject to gastric hydrolysis, while glutathione alone and cysteine are diluted by gastric juice.

There are two forms of Glutathione, the Reduced Glutathione and the Oxidized Glutathione. In order to understand the procedure, we have to understand what NADPH is.

NADPH stands for Nicotinamide Adenine Dinucleotide Phosphate Hydrogen. It is a carrier of Hydrogen. When it gives Hydrogen (-e) with the help of enzymes, it is then called **ADP+**. ADP+ can gain back the Hydrogen with the help of other enzymes. NADPH is made from a chemical reaction called Pentose Phosphate Pathway (PPP) where Glucose is the main component.

From the synthesis above, we have two **Reduced forms of Glutathione**.

2 γ - Glu - Cys - Gly
             |
          SH

Reduced Glutathione has the initials of **GSH**. That is because it has a Sulfhydryl bond (SH). So G stands for Glutathione and SH stands for Sulfhydryl bond.

An oxidant is any oxidizing agent that can destroy bio-molecules as a result of cell death.

If an oxidant comes along, GSH takes a blow and gets oxidized to neutralize the oxidant.

γ - Glu - Cys - Gly
|
S
|
S
|
γ - Glu - Cys - Gly

This is the **Oxidized Glutathione OR Glutathione Disulfide** or **GSSG** (for Glutathione-Sulphur-Sulphur-Glutathione).

What happens if more oxidants come along? That means more GSH are oxidized to GSSG.

If this process continuous on long-term, no GSH will be left to protect us from oxidants.

How is this solved? Our body has found a way to reduce the GSSG with reducing power (NADPH) on GSH with the help of the enzyme Glutathione Reductase.

GSSG + NADPH ⟶ **GSH + NADP+**

Glutathione Reductase

The ratio between GSH and GSSG is what determines cellular toxicity levels. A healthy cell contains about 90% GSH and 10% GSSG. By increasing GSSG, it indicates elevated levels of oxidative stress.

WHAT DEPLETES GLUTATHIONE LEVELS

We can separate the factors that depletes Glutathione levels into internal and external factors.

INTERNAL FACTORS

A. The increasing need for Glutathione for all the properties mentioned above such as in repairing antioxidant, recycling of other antioxidants, protecting the cells for oxidative stress etc.

B. Endogenous toxicity

01	Vaccines	Preservatives like mercury and aluminum that are in high percentage to our vaccines as well as monkey virus SV40 (Simian Virus 40)
02	Chronic conditions	Chronic inflammations that cause exhaustion of organism
03	Old diseases	Diseases that has not been healed in 100% and from time to time they appear depending on the stress
04	Heredity	Having predisposition to any abnormal condition.

EXTERNAL FACTORS

External factors are toxins and harmful substances that we are exposed to on a daily basis, thus requiring greater amounts of Glutathione for their elimination.

Some of these are:

A. Exogenous Toxicity

01	Xenobiotics	Viruses, bacteria, mold, parasites, protozoa
02	Geopathic charge	The anticlockwise spiral energy from the ground causes inflammations
03	Radiation	Microwaves, radio waves, x-rays can cause cancer
04	Electromagnetic field	Electric and magnetic fields are invisible areas of energy that are produced by electricity, which is the movement of electrons, or current through a wire. They also can cause cancer.

05	Shock	Is a life-threatening condition that occurs when the body is not getting enough blood flowing Multiple organs can suffer damage as a result.
06	Heavy metals	Any metallic chemical element that has a relatively high density and is toxic or poisonous at low concentrations. Examples are Mercury, Cadmium, Arsenic, Chromium, Thallium and Lead
07	Pharmaceuticals	Any medicine that is toxic to the body and Glutathione neutralizes it. For example acetaminophen
08	Paint removers & solvents	Methylene chloride, methanol, ethanol, toluene, acetone, mineral spirits (petroleum distilled)
09	Benzopyrenes	Tobacco smoke, barbeque food, fuel exhaust, fuel products and industrial pollutants
10	Pesticides & Herbicides	They block the nervous system of any living organism. Imagine what they do to us.
11	Nitrates & Preservatives	In salami, hot dog, hams, bologna, smoked foods and others
12	Alcohol	When alcohol enters into the body, Glutathione gives tremendous energy to neutralize it and transform it to compounds that can be excreted in the bile or urine.
13	Artificial sweeteners	Aspartame is one of them and is neurotoxin since it is converted to formaldehyde and paralyses the nervous system. Glutathione gives the same energy as in alcohol.
14	Household chemicals	Detergents and fabric softeners, air fresheners, mothballs, mildew removers, cleaners and bleach, lawn and plants fertilizers
15	Houseware chemicals	Non-stick coating of pans and skillets, plastic containers and linings of tin cans and other food packaging.
16	Formaldehyde/styrene	As mentioned above acts as neurotoxin. Found also in photocopiers and toner printers
17	Chlorine	Plays an important role of toxicity when is in treated water

B. Psychosomatic conditions, like depression, anxiety, chronic stress

C. Poor Nutrition resulting to insufficient amount of amino acids, minerals and vitamins, impair Glutathione synthesis and proper function

D. Lack of exercise that leads to the creation of more free radicals to organism

E. Melatonin deficiency. Light pollution (bedside night lights, street lights) lowers glutathione levels because of the suppression of melatonin.

EFFECTS OF GLUTATHIONE DEFICIENCY

Glutathione deficiency occurs when our body is exhausted and unable to produce enough of it to cover all the functions this master tri-peptide performs. This is caused by the factors mentioned in the previous chapter.

Glutathione deficiency can lead to increased oxidative stress, accumulation of more toxins and heavy metals in the body, inability to repair DNA causing autoimmune diseases and cell mutations (cancer), reduced supply of oxygen and nutrients to the cells that results to cell death.

Low Glutathione also means that the prescribed treatments, instead of helping, may actually aggravate the condition because drugs cause further decline in glutathione levels. In HIV patients, the Glutathione levels in their body serves as a measurement indicating how long they can survive.

All chronic and non-chronic conditions are the results of Glutathione deficiency.

01	AUTO-IMMUNE	HIV/AIDS
		Multiple Sclerosis (MS)
		Amyotrophic Lateral Sclerosis (ALS)
		Fibromyalgia
		Diabetes
		Autism
		Parkinson's
		Crohn's Disease
		Autoimmune hepatitis
		Other
02	CANCER	All kinds
03	RESPIRATORY	Asthma
		Allergies
		Bronchitis
		Pneumonia
		Tuberculosis
04	LIVER	Cirrhosis
		Fibrosis
		Wilson's disease
		Viral hepatitis
05	KIDNEY	Inflammation
		Glomerulonephritis

06	DIGESTIVE SYSTEM	Food Intolerance
		Acid Reflux
		Diarrhea
		Others
07	NON-CHRONIC	Flu
		Cold
		Burns
		Trauma

HOW TO GET GLUTATHIONE

Although Reduced Glutathione is a crucial cellular compound, Glutathione in the diet or in the form of supplements does not easily enter inside the cells. Some of the ingested Glutathione that finally reach the cells will be used as separate amino acids where they can help support formation of glutathione inside cells. Increased exposure to damaging environmental chemicals, heavy metals, toxins and medicals, can increase the GSSG level. Supplements of Reduced Glutathione may be used whenever there is an increased need for antioxidant protection and intestinal support of detoxification. Reduced Glutathione is safe to take on a daily basis as long as needed.

1) SULFUR AND PROPER NUTRITION
Here is the diagram of Reduced Glutathione once again:

$$2 \, \gamma - Glu - Cys - Gly$$
$$|$$
$$SH$$

The SH bond in red above equation is the Sulfhydryl Bond. Sulfur is the most important element for the production and proper function of Glutathione.

Dr. Terry Wahls explains very well how she fought Lateral Sclerosis. Here is her story.

> "Dr. Terry Wahls is a clinical professor of medicine at University of Iowa Carver College of Medicine in Iowa City, U.S.A. She teaches internal medicine residents in their primary care clinics. She also does clinical research and have published over 60 peer-reviewed scientific abstracts, posters, and papers. In 2000 she was diagnosed with relapsing remitting multiple sclerosis. In 2003 she was transitioned to secondary progressive multiple sclerosis. She underwent chemotherapy in an attempt to slow the disease and began using a tilt-recline wheelchair because of weakness in back muscle. She made a lot of research -since she was a doctor- to find a solution to the problem but was difficult. She tried supplements but did not succeed. Then she thought, "what if I redesigned my diet so that I was getting those important brain nutrients not from supplements but from the

food I ate?" She realized that synthetic compounds are not biologically the same as what the real food.

She does not mentioned about Glutathione but she does mention about Sulfur. In her diet she emphasizes foods containing sulfur. Like: cauliflower, broccoli, onions, garlic, asparagus, mushrooms, kale, leeks and Brussels sprouts. Among other foods, Dr Terry Wahls had those sulfur containing foods on a daily basis. In 2007 she was in her worst condition. She couldn't even sit in a normal chair. With the help of the paleo diet, progressive exercise program and neuromuscular electrical stimulation, after 3 months she managed to walk with a cane between exam rooms. In six months, she was walking without a cane, and within a year, she was able to get on the bike and start biking again after not having been able to do so for five years.

So according to my experience in practice and what I have studied until now, Sulfur from natural sources, is the #1 substance I could take for consideration".

This means that whatever is the problem, having a natural balance of rich vitamin, mineral, sulfur, protein and fatty acid food, will solve the problem no matter what.

2)   **AMINO ACIDS**

The second important thing to consider is the rest of the structure of Glutathione --- Amino acids. Let's take a look at Amino Acids in general so we can understand and learn what to pay attention to.

20% of the human body is made up of protein. Protein is the body's building block. All of our organs, including the skin, are built from proteins, as are the muscles, hair and nails. Many hormones need proteins to work properly.

Many carriers and enzymes are proteins as well. Protein is, therefore, an essential part of our diet, vital to development, and correct functioning of the body. Protein is particularly important for children and adolescents as they grow and develop into adults, as well as for pregnant women. If our diets do not contain protein, our body would start to break down muscles in order to produce the protein it needs. Remember that the body is good for storing fats and carbohydrates but not proteins.

Protein refers to the type of molecule in food that can be broken down into amino acids. The body needs 22 amino acids.

Why are they called amino acids? All amino acids contain a Carbon atom which forms a bond with an amino group, a carboxyl group, a hydrogen atom and a distinctive R group (R is the rest of the structure of each of the amino acids).

Hence, amino group + carboxyl (acid) group.

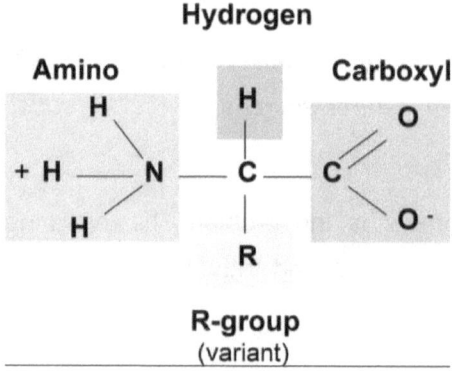

Hydrogen

Amino   **Carboxyl**

R-group
(variant)

According to their biochemical structure they can be divided into seven groups listed below.

	GROUP	DETAILS	AMINO ACIDS
01	ALIPHATIC	Hydrophobic (they resist being in contact with water). Usually are found in the core of the protein.	Glycine, Alanine, Valine, Leucine, Isoleucine, Proline (not so much as the others)
02	AROMATIC	When it contains aromatic ring system	Phenylalanine, Tyrosine, Tryptophan
03	SULFUR	Sulfur containing in their side chains	Cysteine, Methionine, Homocysteine, Taurine

04	HYDROXYLIC	Are polar, uncharged at physiological pH and hydrophilic (they like water because they do not dissolve)	Serine, Threonine
05	BASIC	Their side chains contain Nitrogen and resemble ammonia which is a base	Arginine, Lysine, Histidine
06	ACIDIC	Their sides have Carboxylic acid groups	Aspartate, Glutamate
07	AMIDIC	Containing amide group	Asparagine, Glutamine

Amino acids can be divided into three categories.

(a)The essential

(b) the partially or conditionally essential

(c) the non-essential amino acids.

An essential amino acid is the one that cannot be synthesized by the body, therefore must be supplied by diet. Otherwise, the balance of optimal health is compromised.

The conditionally essential is the amino acid that can be synthesized by the body normally but its synthesis can be limited under patho-physiological conditions. If the system is stressed, out of balance or diseased, these amino acids become essential and must be taken by diet.

The non-essential amino acids are the ones that can be synthesized under physiological and patho-physiological conditions.

Below is the table of the three categories.

ESSENTIAL	PARTIALLY ESSENTIAL	NON-ESSENTIAL
Valine	Glycine	Alanine
Leucine	Cysteine	Asparagine

Isoleucine	Tyrosine	Aspartate
Phenylalanine	Proline	Glutamine
Tryptophan	Glutamine	Glutamate
Threonine	Taurine	Serine
Lysine		
Methionine		
Histidine		
Arginine		

NOTE: The 3 amino acids that are marked in red in the above table are the ones responsible for Glutathione synthesis. Take note that none of them belongs to the essential amino acids. This proves it is important to have good nutrition with natural sulfur and a good mindset.

A. AMINO ACIDS FOR DIRECT PRODUCTION OF GLUTATHIONE

GLUTAMATE: Glutamate is generally acknowledged to be the most important transmitter for normal brain function. Nearly all excitatory neurons in the central nervous system are glutamatergic. It is estimated that over half of all brain synapses release this agent. It belongs to the non-essential group of amino acids and does not cross the blood-brain barrier. It must be synthesized in neurons from local precursors.

The most prevalent glutamate precursor in synaptic terminals is glutamine. Glutamine is released by glial cells and is metabolized to glutamate by the mitochondrial enzyme glutaminase. It also can be synthesized by oxoglutarate in the Tricarboxylic Acid Cycle. Glutamate can be converted to glutamine which is of crucial importance in various biosynthetic processes, transport phenomena, preservation of amino acid balance, and ammonia metabolism. However is also converted to another γ-glutamyl compound of major metabolic significance. It is used together with cysteine and glycine for the biosynthesis of Glutahtione or γ-glutamylcysteinylglycine. All protetin sources are responsible to give glutamate after the degradation of the proteins to amino acids.

GLYCINE: Glycine is produced in the liver from the amino acids serine and threonine but is also abundant in food. It is the smallest of the amino acids. It has several important roles within the body. It is essential for the production of many different acids, including nucleic acids, bile acids, creatine phosphate and porphyrins.

On a broader scale, glycine is involved in the regulation and support of many essential processes. It is closely associated with the central nervous system and the digestive system. Glycine helps with the breakdown of fat by regulating the concentration of bile acids. Glycine is also required for the biosynthesis of Heme.

Heme is a key component of haemoglobin. Haemoglobin is essential in the maintenance of red blood cell integrity and optimal oxygen carrying capacity. Glycine is also an inhibitory neurotransmitter in the central nervous system, which makes it important to help prevent epileptic seizures. It also helps in slowing down the degeneration of muscles (catabolism) since it helps to supply extra Creatine in the body. With the help of Cysteine and Glutamate, they can synthesize Glutathione. Glycine can be found abundant in high protein foods.

CYSTEINE: Cysteine is a sulfur-containing amino acid which for me is the most important amino acid of all. Why? Because of the Sulfur. It can be synthesized from the amino acid Serine. The sulfur is derived from Methionine, which is converted to Homocysteine. Homocysteine and Serine together can synthesize Cysteine.

The level of Cysteine in our body is the limiting factor in how fast we can produce glutathione and how much of it. Cystein is present in all high-protein foods, as well as in plant sources like broccoli, Brussels sprouts, peppers, onions and garlic. However have it in mind that high temperature during cooking, can break down the amide bonds of Cysteine and destroy its bioactivity

B.   AMINO ACIDS FOR INDIRECT PRODUCTION OF GLUTATHIONE

METHIONINE: Cysteine is a sulfur-containing amino acid which is the most important amino acid of all because of the Sulfur. It can be synthesized from the amino acid Serine. The sulfur is derived from Methionine, which is converted to Homocysteine.

Homocysteine and Serine together can synthesize Cysteine. The level of Cysteine in our body is the limiting factor in how fast we can produce glutathione and how much of it. Now as you noticed, Methionine belongs to the essential group of amino acids. There is a possibility, therefore, that with a poor diet, there can be insufficient amount of Cysteine in our body and eventually we will go out of balance.

Food sources for high concentration of Methionine are: Quinoa, buckwheat, sesame seeds, Brazil nuts, meat, fish, eggs and dairy. Another thing to take for consideration is the process of transformation of Methionine into Cysteine. It is a multi-step process and requires the presence of certain enzymes and B-vitamins. This process can be interrupted by liver diseases, impaired metabolism, and others.

Here we have to be injected with substances like N-acetyl-cysteine and Methyl-Sulfonyl-Methane (MSM). These agents, especially the first one, are being used in hospitals to elevate the levels of Cysteine so Glutathione can be synthesized and fight any acute condition.

HOMOCYSTEINE: As mentioned, Methionine is considered to be an essential amino acid. However, in excess, it has been link with many diseases. An 80kg human needs around 1 gram of Methionine per day. The elevated levels of Homocysteine in the blood (homocysteinemia) are associated with elevated oxidative stress. Under healthy conditions, Homocysteine gets converted to either Cysteine or back to Methionine in order not to create damages from too much Homocysteine.

Our body is intelligent and knows how and when to convert these components. What it needs from us is support through proper nutrition and exercise. The reason for this is:

Glycine and Vitamin B6 are essential for converting Homocysteine to Cysteine.

Then more Glycine and Glutamate $\rightleftarrows$ Glutamine are needed to synthesize Glutathione.

If there is not enough Glycine, Cysteine can be converted to Taurine and Sulfate. Vitamin B12, Betaine and Folate help the conversion of Homocysteine to Methionine.

3) WHEY PROTEIN

Milk whey (derived from cow's milk with no hormones and antibiotics in it), contains three highly bioactive proteins: lactoferrin, serum albumin and alpha lactalbumin. These proteins contain exceptional amounts of Cysteine in the form that can enter the cells. Cysteine alone cannot survive in stomach acids unless it is bonded with large proteins. In these proteins, Cysteine is bonded with its Sulfhydryl group to another Cysteine to form Cystine with disulfide bond. Cystine is way much more resistant to stomach acids. Apart from that, whey protein contains the whole gamma of amino acids needed to have a normal balance health. Personally I am a fond of it as I see tremendous results on me and my patients as well. There are a lot of types of Whey Protein, but in order to be effective, it must be kept un-denatured (unheated and unaltered) during the manufacturing process. I prefer isolated enzymatic hydrolyzed whey protein. Some products of high quality whey protein are for example Immunocal of Dr Bounous.

4) ORAL GLUTATHIONE

Glutathione dietary supplements are known as L-glutathione, reduced glutathione or GSH. They come in pills, capsules, tablets, powered and liquid forms, as sublingual drops or slow-melt tablets. However, most people, including medical professionals, are not aware of the fact that these forms may not be very helpful to the body.

Studies: "*Oral glutathione increases tissue glutathione in vivo*", Chemico-Biological Interactions, 1991;80(1):89-97

"*Bioavailability of dietary glutathione: effect on plasma concentration*", The American Journal of Physiology, 1990 Oct; 259(4 Pt 1):G524-9.

Using **liposomal Glutathione** is when the Glutathione molecule is encapsulated in water inside a fat ball that is so small so digestive system "thinks" that is a fat cell so it is not broken down, thus allows it to enter to the bloodstream. The problem is that this molecule starts to be broken down by this phospholipid shield if the supplement sits on a shelf for too long.

5) R-ALPHA LIPOIC ACID (R-ALA)

It is a remarkable antioxidant, partially due to the fact that it is both water soluble and fat soluble. It can cross the blood brain barrier and deactivate free radicals and heavy metals that can create neurodegenerative diseases. R-ALA can increase Glutathione levels by increasing the expression of γ-glutamylcysteine ligase (γ-GCL), the enzyme mentioned above for glutamine-cysteine synthesis. It also increases the cellular uptake of Cysteine.

6) VITAMINS RAISING GLUTATHIONE LEVELS

Vitamin C & E   They both act in a similar way by recycling Glutathione.

Vitamin B1 &   Both maintain Glutathione and its enzymes in their active
B2   form.

Vitamin B2	Helps convert amino acids into proteins
Vitamin B6	Crucial for the metabolism of Homocysteine into Cysteine
Vitamin B9	Helps in giving Cysteine to Glutathione and is not converted back to Hmocysteine
Vitamin B12	Helps indirectly by helping in the production of red blood cells

7) ELEMENTS RAISING GLUTATHIONE LEVELS

Selenium	Together with Vitamin E they elevate the level of activated Glutathione
Magnesium	It is responsible for the proper functioning of enzyme γ-glutamyl transpeptidase mentioned above
Zinc	Not proper levels in the body can reduce the level of active intracellular Glutathione. The ratio of copper and zinc must be 7:1. A lot of foods can contain a lot of copper but no zinc. Sources like grains, nuts, seeds, beans and chocolate. We need to balance those 2 elements because lower zinc can lead also to hyperactivity, depression and enhance autism as well as any other disease because of the low levels of Glutathione.

SUMMARY

In order to understand the power of Glutathione, just remember the 3 powerful "musts" that will help you live longer, healthier and wealthier:

1. Nutrition (including greens and whey protein)

2. Daily Exercise

3. Mindset and daily meditation.

For any questions regarding Glutathione, do not hesitate to contact me at: drneohealth@gmail.com

REFERENCES

"*Glutathione (GSH) - Your Body's Most Powerful Protector*" Dr. Jimmy Gtuman MD, FACEP, 3rd edition

"*The Master Antioxidant - Glutathione*" Jeffrey Sutton

"*The Mother of all Antioxidants - Glutathione*" Joey Lott

"*Glutathione - its role in cancer and anticancer therapy*" Dr. Jimmy Gutman, MD, FACEP

"*Breakthrough in cell-defense - how to benefit from the REAL Glutathione Revolution*" Dr Allan C. Somarsall, PhD, MD, Dr Gustavo Bounous, MD, FRCS (C)

"*Avoiding the First Cause of Death: Can we live longer and better?*" Wulf Droge

"Biochemistry" Stryer. Fourth Edition

ABOUT THE AUTHOR

Dr. Neophytos Neophytou, or simply Dr. Neo, is a multi-faceted man who is successful in the many endeavors he engages in. He is a businessman, an author, a sportsman, a family physician, a veterinary surgeon, and a holistic practitioner rolled into one.

His career as a veterinary doctor started in 2005 when he earned his diploma in Veterinary Medicine from the Agricultural University of Wroclaw, Poland. Five years later, he became a full-pledge veterinary surgeon upon completion of his Post Graduate course in Veterinary Surgery in the same university. However, his love for animals started much earlier during his youth when his family put up a pig farm business.

Dr. Neo's concern for the health and welfare of animals went beyond animals to include the whole humanity. This led him to further his studies by enrolling at the College of Naturopathic Medicine UK via the Neo-Hippocrates Natural Therapies in Cyprus.

In 2014, he earned his two diplomas both for Naturopathic and Homeopathic Medicines from the Neo-Hippocrates Natural Therapies in Cyprus. In the same year, besides taking up Energy Healing courses in Cyprus, he also studied Electromagnetic Waves Diagnosis and Healing at the Deta Elis Russian Institute and MLM.

Equipped with all these knowledge, Dr. Neo embarked in his life-long dream of caring both for humans and animals as a veterinarian, a family physician, and a holistic health practitioner.

In his medical practice, Dr. Neo gives a special attention on detoxification. He believes that the detoxification of organisms and the neutralization of their emotional state from cell memories are the most powerful weapons in combating diseases. He has been very successful with Glutathione in detoxifying patients and has successfully cured diseases which conventional medicine fails to resolve.

ABOUT THE BOOK

This book, "A Secret for A Longer and Better Life", points out some facts about this significant component of our nutrients known as Glutathione. It makes us aware of the essential role it plays in the proper functioning of our body. We learn to appreciate and value its contribution to a healthier and happier life.

www.ingramcontent.com/pod-product-compliance
Lightning Source LLC
Chambersburg PA
CBHW051406280526
45784CB00007B/3118